THAI MAS

The Essential Guide To Thai Massage: Understanding Step-By-Step Manual For Mindful Bodywork

NUEL NENJI

Contents

Introductory

Thai massage, alternatively referred to as Thai yoga massage or Thai Nuad Boran, is an ancient Thai therapeutic modality. It is a bodywork technique that integrates acupressure, traditional massage, and yoga.

The underlying principle of this practice is that energy traverses the body via distinct pathways known as "sen" or "meridians," and by manipulating these energy lines, one can achieve enhanced physical and mental health.

Crucial components of Thai massage consist of:

• A sequence of passive poses resembling those found in yoga are incorporated into Thai massage in order to increase range of motion, flexibility, and relaxation.

• Utilizing their palms, thumbs, elbows, knees, and feet, the therapist applies acupressure to specific points along the energy lines of the body. This is comparable to acupuncture in principle, but it does not involve the insertion of needles.

• Joint mobilization: Thai massage incorporates joint manipulation and mobilization techniques, which enhance flexibility and alignment.

• Thai massage aims to achieve an energetic equilibrium within the body by stimulating a harmonious passage along its numerous energy pathways.

• Breath awareness and mindfulness: During the session, both the practitioner and the recipient employ deep breathing and mindfulness techniques, which serve to augment the overall therapeutic encounter.

The mat is typically laid out on the floor during Thai massage, and the recipient remains completely clothed. The massage is frequently characterized as an interactive and dynamic form of bodywork in which both the therapist and the recipient collaborate to attain the intended results.

An overall sense of well-being and relaxation, as well as improved circulation, increased vitality, and enhanced flexibility, may be among the benefits of Thai massage.

It is imperative to acknowledge that although Thai massage can provide advantages for a considerable number of people, it may not be appropriate for all, particularly those who have specific medical conditions. It is recommended that individuals prior to undergoing any type of massage therapy, including Thai massage, consult with a healthcare professional.

CHAPTER ONE
Fundamentals Of Thai Massage

Thai massage is guided in its practice by a number of fundamental principles. These principles comprise the theoretical foundation of the therapy as well as the methodologies employed throughout a session. The following are several foundational tenets of Thai massage:

• Sen Lines: "Sen" lines, which are comparable to the energy meridians in traditional Chinese medicine, form the basis of Thai massage. It is hypothesized that vital energy (referred to as "lom" or "prana") flows through these sen lines. Achieving energy flow balance and unblocking is the fundamental objective of Thai massage, which involves the manipulation of these energy lines.

• Thai massage integrates passive poses reminiscent of yoga in order to enhance flexibility and facilitate the circulation of energy. Frequently rhythmic and arranged in a fluid sequence, the stretches resemble a dance performed by the practitioner and the recipient.

• The therapist administers pressure to specific acupressure points along the sen lines with their feet, hands, thumbs, elbows, and knees. The primary objectives of this acupressure technique are to alleviate tension, enhance energy circulation, and rectify bodily imbalances.

• Thai massage consists of joint mobilization and compression in addition to fingertip manipulation and soft tissue mobilization. This facilitates improved flexibility, decreased muscle tension, and increased circulation.

• Breath Awareness: During the session, both the therapist and the recipient are encouraged to engage in mindful, steady breathing. Conscious respiration facilitates the circulation of energy and aids in relaxation.

• Metta (Loving-Kindness): The principle of "metta," which represents loving-kindness, is frequently integrated into Thai massage. It is recommended that practitioners adopt a compassionate and mindful demeanor when performing massage, thereby establishing a therapeutic atmosphere that transcends the mere execution of physical techniques.

• Traditional Thai massage places significant emphasis on the practitioner exhibiting four attitudes that are considered fundamental to the practice: compassion, equanimity, pleasure, and mindfulness. These attitudes facilitate the recipient's holistic and therapeutic experience.

• Thai massage is flexible with regard to the comfort level and requirements of the recipient. Encouragement of communication between the client and the practitioner ensures a comfortable and effective massage.

Thai massage is an interactive and dynamic modality of bodywork that places equal emphasis on the energetic and physical dimensions of harmony. A holistic approach to health is frequently regarded as one that considers the body, mind, and spirit.

The Advantages Of Thai Massage

Thai massage provides an extensive array of prospective physical and mental benefits. The following are a few of the frequently noted benefits:

• Stretching and yoga-like motions incorporated into Thai massage can assist in enhancing flexibility through the stimulation of various muscle groups and joints.

• Enhanced Circulation: The integration of acupressure, compression, and stretching techniques within Thai massage has the potential to augment blood flow, thereby potentially resulting in an all-around improvement in circulation.

• Thai massage, similar to other types of massage, has the potential to induce relaxation and alleviate tension. By combining mindful respiration with physical manipulation, one can experience a heightened state of tranquility.

• Muscle Tension Relief: Thai massage's acupressure and compression techniques can assist in the release of muscle tension, resulting in a decrease in pain and discomfort.

• Thai massage integrates joint mobilization techniques, which have the potential to enhance joint functionality and alleviate stiffness.

• Energy Harmonization: Thai massage, which is predicated on the notion of sen lines and energy circulation, endeavors to harmonize the body's energy, thereby potentially fostering holistic health.

• Thai massage incorporates a series of stretches and movements that potentially enhance joint mobility and facilitate an expanded range of motion.

• Promoting a sense of harmony, the emphasis on breath awareness and mindfulness during a Thai massage session can assist in establishing a more robust mind-body connection.

• An increase in joint mobility and the alleviation of muscle tension are two potential benefits of Thai massage that could lead to an improvement in posture.

• Discharge of Emotional Tension: Thai massage has been reported by some practitioners and recipients to assist in the discharge of emotional stress and tension in addition to physical tension.

• Enhanced Immune System: The potential benefits of Thai massage on the immune system may derive from the associated relaxation and stress reduction.

• Better Sleep Quality: The relaxation that Thai massage elicits in numerous individuals has been found to contribute to enhanced sleep.

It is imperative to acknowledge that individual Thai massage experiences may differ, and the efficacy of the treatment is contingent upon several factors, including the practitioner's expertise, the recipient's health status, and personal inclinations.

Moreover, although Thai massage offers a multitude of advantages, it might not be appropriate for all individuals, particularly those who are afflicted with specific medical conditions.

It is advisable for individuals to seek the advice of a healthcare professional prior to engaging in any type of massage therapy.

CHAPTER TWO
A Comprehension Of Thai Massage

Comprehending Thai massage necessitates an awareness of its inception, fundamentals, methodologies, and prospective advantages. The following is a breakdown:

1. In origin:

• Thai massage is a therapeutic practice that originates from traditional Thai medicine, an amalgamation of Ayurvedic, Chinese, and yogic principles.

Energies and Sen Lines:

• Energy transmission and the notion of "sen" lines are fundamental to comprehending the operation of Thai massage. Let us take a closer look:

1. Sentimental Lines:

• Sen lines are bodily energy channels or pathways through which it is believed that life force energy, also referred to as "lom" or "prana," circulates.

• The number of sen lines in the human body is estimated to be around 72,000; however, Thai massage frequently places emphasis on the primary ten.

• Concentrate on Ten Sen Lines: Thai massage frequently targets the principal ten sen lines, which are significant energy channels linked to a multitude of physiological and energetic processes.

2. Energy Transmission:

• Thai massage is designed to restore equilibrium to the energy circulation within the sen lines. There is a belief that energy stagnation or obstruction can result in physical discomfort, agony, or illness.

- Unblocking Energy: Thai massage practitioners employ various techniques, including acupressure and stretching, to facilitate the release of blockages in the sen lines, thereby enhancing the unrestricted passage of energy.

- Thai massage employs a holistic methodology that encompasses the physical and energetic dimensions of the human being. The objective is to establish equilibrium and harmony across the complete system.

3. Utilizing Sensation Lines in Thai Massage:

• Practitioners utilize their palms, thumbs, elbows, knees, and feet to apply pressure to particular acupressure points along the sen lines. Comparable to acupressure as practiced in traditional Chinese medicine.

• Thai massage incorporates stretching and yoga-like movements into its technique with the intention of stimulating and opening the sen lines, thereby facilitating a harmonious and equilibrium of energy circulation.

• Joint mobilization is a therapeutic approach utilized to rectify energy imbalances and enhance the circulation of energy within and in the vicinity of the joints.

4. Regarding philosophy:

• Energetic Harmony: Thai massage is founded upon the principle that the harmonious circulation of energy within the body is intrinsically linked to both physical and mental wellness.

• Prevention and Maintenance: In addition to its application in resolving specific concerns, Thai massage is frequently employed as a preventive and maintenance modality to facilitate the uninterrupted flow of energy and uphold general well-being.

Gaining comprehension of sen lines and energy flow within the context of Thai massage offers valuable insights into the practice's holistic essence, underscoring the interdependence of physical, mental, and energetic dimensions of wellness. The therapeutic objectives of Thai massage revolve around the manipulation of sen lines, which are intended to restore equilibrium and vitality to the recipient.

Traditional Thai Massage Method Nuad Bo Rarn

Therapeutic Nuad Bo Rarn, also referred to as Traditional Thai Massage, originates from the ancient medicinal traditions of Thailand. The English translation of the appellation "Nuad Bo Rarn" is "traditional massage" or "ancient massage."

A combination of acupressure, yoga-like stretches, joint mobilization, and energy harmonizing comprise this method.

A synopsis of the fundamental components of Nuad Bo Rarn follows:

1. Setting and Garments:

• Thai massage, in contrast to certain alternative massage modalities, generally entails the complete cling of the recipient to the body. It is advisable to wear comfortable, loose apparel in order to facilitate unrestricted motion throughout the stretches and manipulations.

• Mat on the Floor: The massage is customarily performed on a mat that is positioned on the floor, which facilitates the practitioner's mobility and enables the execution of diverse stretches and manipulations.

2. The Relationship Between Sen lines and energy flow:

• The Nuad Bo Rarn practice entails the manipulation of the sen lines, which are purported energy pathways that traverse the entirety of the body. Ten major sen lines are targeted throughout a traditional Thai massage.

• Energy Balancing: The objective is to achieve a state of equilibrium and harmony in one's well-being by regulating the flow of energy along these sen lines.

3. Compression and Acupressure:

• Acupressure Points: Practitioners apply pressure to designated acupressure points along the sen lines using their palms, thumbs, elbows, knees, and feet. This facilitates energy transmission and aids in the release of tension.

• Compression Techniques: To promote relaxation and enhanced circulation, the therapist may employ rhythmic compression, gentle swaying, palm presses, and gentle rocking to target the muscles and soft tissues.

4. Prandial Stretches:

• Passive stretching, a characteristic that sets Nuad Bo Rarn apart, is its incorporation of yoga-like movements. Assisting the recipient in assuming a variety of stretching and mobilization positions for joints and muscle groups.

• Range of Motion: The objective of these stretches is to augment the individual's overall range of motion, improve flexibility, and enhance joint mobility.

5. Joint Activation:

• Moderate Manipulation: To enhance the flexibility and

functionality of the joints, Thai massage incorporates moderate joint mobilization techniques. This may prove to be especially advantageous in mitigating tension and fostering improved alignment.

6. Breath Observation:

• Mindful Breathing: During the session, both the practitioner and the recipient are encouraged to engage in profound, mindful breathing. Conscious respiration facilitates the overall therapeutic experience and promotes relaxation.

7. Holistic Methodology:

• The Body-Mind-Spirit Connection: Nuad Bo Rarn is regarded as a comprehensive practice that attends to the energetic and mental dimensions of well-being in addition to the physical body. Its purpose is to encourage harmony and equilibrium in the body-mind-spirit connection.

Traditional Thai Massage, or Nuad Bo Rarn, is renowned for its comprehensive approach to promoting health and overall well-being. By integrating acupressure, stretching, and energy work, this therapeutic bodywork approach distinguishes itself as an all-encompassing and distinctive method of restoring equilibrium and vitality.

CHAPTER THREE
The Distinction Between Western And Thai Massage

Western massage and Thai massage are two discrete modalities of bodywork that diverge in terms of their underlying philosophies, methodologies, and cultural impact. Several significant distinctions exist between the two:

1. The Philosophy and History:

• Thai massage, also known as Nuad Bo Rarn, has its origins in Thailand. Its foundations lie in traditional Thai medicine, while also integrating components from Ayurveda, yoga, and Chinese medicine. Achieving energy balance within the organism, it emphasizes the notion of sen lines (energy pathways).

• Western massage comprises a diverse array of techniques, including sports massage, deep tissue massage, and Swedish massage. Constantly emphasizing physiological responses and anatomical structures, its objectives are to promote relaxation, enhance circulation, and alleviate muscle tension.

2. Setting and Garments:

• Thai massage is commonly conducted while the recipient is completely clad, donning loose-fitting and comfortable garments. Stretches and manipulations are frequently performed by the practitioner using bodyweight and leverage while seated on a mat on the floor.

• Western massage is typically executed while the recipient is clothed in linens or towels and undressed to their preferred degree of comfort. The massage is frequently performed on a massage platform.

3. Methods of Technique:

• Thai massage incorporates a variety of therapeutic techniques, including energy harmonizing methods, passive yoga-like stretches, joint mobilization, and acupressure. As pressure is exerted along the sen lines, a series of stretches are performed while the recipient is guided.

• Western massage incorporates a variety of techniques, which differ depending on the modality but frequently comprise petrissage (kneading), friction, effleurage (long, gliding strokes), and tapotement (percussive movements). A prevalent modality in the West, deep tissue massage targets deeper strata of muscle tissue.

4. Sensing and Energy Lines:

• Thai massage is founded upon the fundamental principles of sen lines and the need to restore equilibrium to the energy flow within the body. Acupressure is applied to particular points along the sen lines in order to facilitate the flow of energy and eliminate obstructions.

• Western massage differs in that although certain modalities may integrate energy principles, the primary objective is frequently the treatment of bodily organs, muscular systems, and blood flow, with little attention paid to energy lines.

5. Client Involvement:

• Thai massage frequently elicits active engagement from the recipient as the practitioner guides them through a series of stretches and positions. This is a more interactive session.

• In Western massage, the recipient generally assumes a more passive position by reclining on the massage table as the therapist executes the various techniques.

6. Objective of the Session:

• Thai massage endeavors to achieve energy balance, enhance flexibility, and foster holistic well-being. It is regarded as a holistic method because it considers the body, mind, and spirit.

• In Western massage, objectives may encompass pain relief, relaxation, tension mitigation, and targeted attention to specific muscular concerns. Frequently, it corresponds with a greater emphasis on biomechanics and physiology.

7. Length of the Session:

• Thai massage sessions frequently extend from 1.5 to 2 hours in length, providing sufficient time to incorporate the holistic techniques of acupressure and stretching.

• Western Massage: Depending on the modality and the client's preferences, sessions typically last between 30 and 90 minutes.

Thai massage and Western massage each offer distinct advantages, and individuals may opt for one over the other according to personal inclinations, health objectives, or cultural factors. Communicating with the massage therapist is crucial in order to ensure that the selected modality is in accordance with the individual's requirements and expectations.

Precautions In Advance Of A Thai Massage

A number of factors must be taken into account prior to a Thai massage in order to guarantee a pleasant and comfortable experience. The following are some suggestions:

1. Put on comfortable attire:

• Thai massage is commonly administered while the recipient is completely clad. Put on comfortable, loose-fitting attire that facilitates unrestricted motion. Avoid wearing restrictive apparel or tight jeans.

2. Dialogue involving the therapist:

• Please inform the therapist of any health concerns or specific issues that you would like to have addressed throughout the session.

• Please communicate any injuries, medical conditions, or sensitive areas to the therapist.

3. Make an Early Arrival:

• One should arrive slightly prior to the massage session in order to complete any required documentation and to allow for some relaxation time.

4. A Light Meal Prior to the Session:

• It is advisable to restrict hefty meals immediately preceding the massage. It is advisable to consume a light snack or supper a few hours prior to the session.

5. Remove accessories and jewelry:

• Prior to the session, remove any jewelry, timepieces, or accessories that may potentially disrupt the massage techniques.

6. Expression of Preferences:

• Please communicate your preferences to the therapist concerning pressure, areas of focus, and any particular techniques that may or may not be suitable for you.

• Promote frank communication throughout the session. If the pressure becomes excessive or if you experience any distress, please communicate this to the therapist.

7. Specify Regarding Pregnancy or Health Concerns:

• Pregnancy and any other pertinent health concerns should be communicated to the therapist beforehand. There may be certain adjustments that are necessary for expectant women.

8. Conscious Breathing:

• Engage in mindful respiration both prior to and throughout the session. Slow, deep breaths can facilitate connection with the therapeutic experience and promote relaxation.

9. Intentions of Relaxation:

• Originate a state of relaxation and release of tension throughout the session. Place your complete reliance on the therapist's expertise and permit yourself to completely benefit from the massage.

10. Sufficient hydration:

• Stay hydrated by consuming copious amounts of water prior to and following the massage. Toxins can be eliminated from the musculature through massage, and hydration aids in the body's natural detoxification.

11. Pre-Massage Strategies:

• Schedule a period of relaxation and repose following the massage. It is advisable to refrain from engaging in physically demanding activities immediately after the session in order to facilitate the body's absorption of the therapeutic effects.

12. Appreciation and esteem:

• Initiate the session by exhibiting an attitude of appreciation and deference towards the practitioner. Fostering an atmosphere of positivity and receptiveness may enhance the overall harmony of an encounter.

Bear in mind the criticality of communication with the massage therapist. By customizing the session to suit your particular requirements, they will guarantee your complete comfort during the entire procedure.

By adhering to these guidelines, you can maximize your Thai massage experience.

CHAPTER FOUR
Thai Massage Methods

A variety of Thai massage techniques are employed to promote energy balance, tension release, and general health. The following are essential Thai massage techniques:

1. Thumbing and Palming:

• The practitioner employs their palms, fingertips, and thumbs to exert rhythmic pressure on designated areas along the sen lines of the body. Similar to acupressure, this method is intended to clear energy obstructions.

2. Line of Sentiment Tracing:

• The therapist facilitates the unimpeded circulation of energy throughout the body by applying pressure and stretches along the sen lines, which are pathways of energy.

3. Yoga-Like Stretching and Movements:

• Thai massage is distinguished in part by the use of inert stretching techniques. While guiding the recipient into a series of yoga-like positions, the therapist tenderly stretches and mobilizes various muscle groups and joints using their body, hands, and feet.

4. Joint Activation:

• In order to enhance joint functionality and flexibility, light joint manipulation and movement are integrated. This method has the potential to alleviate rigidity and increase range of motion.

5. The compression process:

• Compression is accomplished by utilizing force to contract muscles and tender tissues. The therapist may apply pressure and alleviate tension in particular areas using their feet, palms, elbows, knees, or knees.

6. Rhythmic and rocking motion:

• The practitioner may induce a state of fluidity and relaxation through the use of rhythmic movements and swaying motions. This technique aids in providing the recipient with a tranquil and meditative experience.

7. Fingers on the palm and circular motions:

• Circular motions and palm pressures are utilized in order to induce a sensation of warmth in the treated areas, promote blood circulation, and relax muscles.

8. Work on the Breath and Mindfulness:

• Both the practitioner and the recipient participate in synchronized, deep breathing exercises with the intention of augmenting relaxation and mindfulness. Breathing deliberately is an essential component of the Thai massage experience.

9. Thai Foot Hygiene:

• Thai massage may also incorporate specialized foot techniques, in addition to its bodily targets. The application of reflexology and massage techniques to the feet serves to enhance energy circulation and foster holistic health.

10. Point-of-trigger therapy:

• The therapist may identify particular trigger points, areas of muscle tension, or sensitive regions and apply pressure to those areas. This may assist in pain relief and tension discharge.

11. Energy Equilibrium:

• Thai massage operates on the principle of energy balance within the body. Methods are implemented with the explicit purpose of fostering equilibrium and concordance within the energy conduits.

12. Supplementary Herbal Compress:

• In certain Thai massage sessions, heated bundles of botanicals known as herbal compresses may be utilized as application pads. Heat and herbal aromas potentially have additional therapeutic benefits in addition to promoting relaxation.

It is essential to note that Thai massage is frequently tailored to the requirements and preferences of the individual. Practitioners have the ability to modify techniques in order to target particular concerns or address specific issues.

Effective communication between the clinician and the recipient is crucial for a productive and comfortable session.

Body Mechanics For Practitioners Of Thai Massage

In order to prevent self-injury and increase the efficacy of the massage, Thai massage practitioners must observe correct body mechanics. The following are essential body mechanics principles for Thai massage practitioners:

1. Sustain a Stable Foundation:

• Develop a stable foundation by positioning your ankles shoulder-width apart. Equally distribute your body weight across both feet.

2. Supine at the Knees:

• Avoid bending at the waist when conducting techniques that require forward bending, such as stretches or applying pressure. Instead, bend at the knees. This contributes to lower spine protection.

3. Employ Your Body Mass:

• Pressure is frequently applied through the utilization of body weight in Thai massage. Particularly when performing compressions, utilize your complete body to apply pressure as opposed to relying solely on your upper body strength.

4. Activate Your Core:

• Engage your core muscles in order to maintain appropriate posture and support your spine. This reduces the burden on your back and assists in the distribution of the workload.

5. Adequate Posture:

• Maintain a neutral and upright spine position. Prevent yourself from slouching or curving your shoulders. In addition to preventing strain, proper posture facilitates enhanced energy circulation throughout the massage.

6. Employ the Legs and Hips:

• Lengthen and incorporate the legs and pelvis into stretches and movements. This facilitates a more regulated and seamless implementation of methodologies.

7. Efficient Transitions:

• It is important to develop the ability to transition between techniques seamlessly. Avoid abrupt or jerky motions, as they may cause the recipient discomfort and strain your own muscles.

8. Adjust to Variable Heights:

• To optimize one's posture and approach, it is essential to consider the recipient's height. This guarantees that appropriate body mechanics can be maintained irrespective of the size or shape of the recipient.

9. Preserve Adaptability:

• Stretch and maintain your own flexibility on a regular basis. This is essential for performing the required yoga-like movements and poses in Thai massage without subjecting your body to unnecessary strain.

10. Interactions Regarding the Recipient:

• Inquire with the recipient regarding their level of comfort, particularly in regards to stretching. Ascertain that they are in a calm state and devoid of any pain or discomfort.

11. Employ Correct Hand Positions:

• Sustain appropriate hand and forearm alignment in order to mitigate strain. To prevent overextension, be mindful of your hand positions during techniques such as thumb pressure.

12. Endurance and Temporality:

• Maintain endurance throughout the session by keeping your pace. By consistently conditioning and practicing, one can increase stamina and prevent fatigue.

13. Consistent Self-Care:

• One should incorporate self-care practices, such as stretching exercises and massages, into their daily regimens in order to safeguard against burnout and injury.

14. Persisting in Education:

• Maintain a comprehensive understanding of appropriate body mechanics and contemplate continuous education in order to enhance your skills and acquire knowledge of novel methodologies that may be more physiologically sustainable.

By integrating these fundamental principles of body mechanics into their therapeutic approach, Thai massage practitioners can ensure that their clients have comfortable and efficacious sessions, all the while protecting their own physical welfare.

CHAPTER FIVE
Thai Massage Intunements

Sequences of Thai massage pertain to the precise combination and arrangement of techniques employed throughout a massage session.

Although each practitioner may employ unique techniques and variations, the fundamental principles of Thai massage are rooted in recurring sequences. The following is an overview of the sequence of a traditional Thai massage.

1. Centering and Opening:

• Frequently, the session commences with the practitioner and recipient sharing a moment of connection and centering. A brief meditation, deep breathing, or gentle swaying motion may be required.

2. Performing a Foot Massage:

• The therapist may commence the session by performing a foot massage, employing methods including palm strokes and thumb pressures to soothe the feet and promote the circulation of energy.

3. Line of Sentiment Tracing:

• The therapist employs circular motions, palming, and thumbing, to trace the energy pathways along the sen lines, which are located on the back, thighs, and arms. This facilitates the body's readiness for more strenuous stretches.

4. Stretched Legs:

• The recipient is led through a succession of passive leg stretches. In order to enhance flexibility and alleviate tension, these stretches may encompass light rotation, bending, and tugging.

5. Positions on the Side:

• While the recipient lies on their side, the therapist proceeds with stretch exercises and sensitization techniques, with particular emphasis on the lower limbs and hips.

6. Back Exercise Methods:

• The practitioner applies techniques to the back, including thumb presses, palm presses, and mild stretches, to the recipient while they are on their stomach. These techniques are intended to alleviate tension in the shoulders and back.

7. Engaging in Prone Stretching:

• The therapist places the recipient in a variety of prone positions so that stretching and manipulations can be performed on the shoulders, hips, and back.

8. Supine Position Methods:

• While the recipient is in a relaxed reclining position, the therapist performs pressure on the upper back, shoulders, and neck. Stretching and moderate compressions may be required.

9. A Head and Neck Massage:

• The clinician may employ neck stretches and a light head massage as therapeutic techniques to alleviate neck tension and facilitate relaxation.

10. Scalp and Facial Massage:

• In order to promote relaxation and offer a calming conclusion to the session, a mild face and scalp massage may be performed to conclude the session.

11. Grounding and Closing:

• The session concludes with a concluding ritual that restores the recipient to a state of equilibrium through deep breathing, a moment of gratitude, or a gentle rocking motion.

Notably, the sequence may differ depending on the practitioner's approach, the requirements of the recipient, and the particular objectives of the session.

Proficient Thai massage practitioners have the ability to tailor sequences according to specific elements, including the recipient's health, personal preferences, and any particular concerns they wish to target.

Effective communication is essential between the Thai massage practitioner and the recipient in order to guarantee a customized and successful session.

Thai Prenatal Massage

Prenatal Thai massage is an adapted variant of the traditional Thai massage style, designed to cater to the unique requirements and safety concerns of expectant women.

The intervention integrates non-invasive and encouraging strategies to attend to the distinct physiological and psychological transformations that transpire throughout the course of pregnancy. The following are essential elements and considerations of prenatal Thai massage:

1. Consultation and Communication:

• Prior to the commencement of the session, the therapist engages in an extensive consultation with the expectant woman in order to gain a comprehensive understanding of her medical background, any existing complications, and any particular concerns she may have. Effective communication is essential for a comfortable and secure experience.

2. Appropriate Positioning:

• Prenatal Thai massage frequently involves the client in a semi-reclined or side-lying position, bolsters and pillows providing support. This positioning aids in the alleviation of abdominal pressure and guarantees the expectant individual's safety and comfort.

3. Mild motions and stretches:

• The massage consists of light stretching and motions that are appropriate for women who are expectant. The therapist employs modified techniques in order to prevent abdominal and lower back strain.

4. Concentrate on Reducing Stress and Relaxation:

• Prenatal Thai massage prioritizes the promotion of relaxation and the alleviation of tension. Methods have been developed with the intention of reducing edema and lower back pain, which are common discomforts associated with pregnancy, and to soothe the nervous system.

5. Joint Activation:

• A series of light joint mobilization techniques may be utilized to alleviate joint stiffness and discomfort, particularly in the shoulder and hip regions.

6. Points of Pressure and Energy Work:

• The therapist may target particular pressure points in order to alleviate prevalent pregnancy-related symptoms such as fatigue, migraines, or nausea. The primary emphasis is on fostering holistic wellness and equilibrium.

7. Breath Observation:

• Professionals frequently recommend deep breathing exercises as a means to assist expectant women in unwinding and maintaining awareness of their breath during the session.

8. Modifications to Adapt to Each Trimester:

• Depending on the stage of pregnancy of the individual, the massage may be modified. There may be adjustments to specific techniques and positions as the pregnancy advances.

9. Avoidance of Particular Regions:

• In order to prioritize the safety of the mother and the infant, it is customary to avoid or exercise extra caution when treating areas such as the abdomen and inner thighs.

10. Comfort & Hydration Breaks:

• It is advisable for pregnant women to maintain adequate hydration, and the therapist may provide comfort intervals as required. It is imperative that the participant express any unease or apprehensions that may arise throughout the session.

11. Expertise Training:

• It is imperative that prenatal Thai massage practitioners possess specialized training in prenatal massage techniques and a comprehensive knowledge of the physiological transformations and factors to be taken into account during pregnancy.

It is imperative that expectant mothers consult their healthcare provider prior to undergoing any type of prenatal massage, including Thai massage. Additionally, to ensure a safe and supportive experience, they should retain the services of a certified and seasoned massage therapist who specializes in prenatal care.

Thai Massage With Runners

Incorporating Thai massage into an athlete's recuperation and overall wellness regimen may prove to be beneficial.

By integrating a sequence of joint mobilization, compression, and stretching exercises, this regimen can alleviate muscle tension, enhance flexibility, and encourage relaxation. In the following ways, Thai massage can be especially beneficial for athletes:

1. Enhanced adaptability:

• A variety of muscle groups and joints are targeted with passive stretching techniques in Thai massage. This may potentially enhance flexibility, a critical attribute for athletes seeking to optimize performance and mitigate the likelihood of sustaining injuries.

2. Increasing the Range of Motion:

• Thai massage's joint mobilization and stretching techniques contribute to an increase in joint flexibility and overall range of motion. This can be particularly advantageous for athletes engaged in activities that demand an extensive repertoire of motions.

3. Analgesic Muscle Tension:

• Muscle tension is alleviated through the integration of acupressure and compression techniques within Thai massage. This can be especially beneficial for athletes who, as a result of vigorous physical activity, develop muscle tension and knots.

4. Preventing Injuries By:

• Regular Thai massage has the potential to aid in injury prevention through the mitigation of tension in injury-prone areas, correction of muscular imbalances, and promotion of proper alignment.

5. More Rapid Recovery:

• Thai massage reduces muscle fatigue and enhances blood circulation, thereby facilitating post-exercise recovery. Thai massage techniques have the potential to accelerate the recuperation process following strenuous physical exertion.

6. Encouragement of Relaxation:

• Thai massage's meditative and soothing qualities can assist athletes in attaining a state of physical and mental relaxation. Reducing stress is critical for optimal physical and mental health, as well as for enhanced performance.

7. Enhanced Perfusion:

• Thai massage's periodic compressions and stretches have the potential to improve blood circulation, facilitating the transportation of nutrients and oxygen to the muscles while also supporting waste elimination.

8. Tackling Particular Concerns:

• Particularly troublesome areas for athletes include the shoulders, hip flexors, and hamstrings. Thai massage has the capacity to be customized in order to target and alleviate these particular concerns.

9. Harmonizing Energy:

• The therapeutic approach, which is grounded in the notion of energy lines in Thai massage, endeavors to restore equilibrium to the energy circulation within the body. By adopting this comprehensive approach, athletes can enhance their overall vitality and well-being.

10. Enhanced Physical Awareness:

• Thai massage promotes body awareness and mindfulness. Individuals who are more physiologically attuned may possess the ability to detect and resolve issues with their bodies prior to their progression into more serious complications.

11. Adaptation to Sport-Specific Requirements:

• Proficient Thai massage practitioners possess the ability to tailor sessions in order to cater to the unique requirements and pressures of various sports, thereby guaranteeing that the treatment is in accordance with the training and performance objectives of the athlete.

It is imperative for athletes to maintain open lines of communication with their massage therapist regarding their training regimen, particular areas of concern, injuries, or conditions.

It is recommended that athletes seek guidance from their healthcare professionals prior to integrating any novel bodywork technique, such as Thai massage, into their wellness regimen.

Summary

Thai massage, which originated in Thailand and has since garnered international renown, is a multifaceted and holistic therapeutic practice.

It integrates acupressure, passive stretching, joint mobilization, and energy balancing, all of which are derived from traditional Thai medicine, with the aim of fostering both physical and mental wellness. The underlying principle of the practice is sen lines, which are energy pathways through which vital life force circulates.

Thai massage provides a multitude of potential advantages, encompassing enhanced circulation, improved flexibility, alleviation of muscle tension, joint mobilization, and a comprehensive approach to restoring energy balance to the body. By prioritizing respiratory awareness and mindfulness, one can cultivate a more profound mind-body connection.

Knowledge of Thai massage's principles, techniques, and the significance of sen lines and energy transmission are essential for comprehension. The practice has been modified to serve a multitude of objectives, such as providing assistance to athletes, addressing particular health issues, and accommodating expectant women.

In order to be prepared for a Thai massage session, one must don comfortable attire, engage in open communication with the therapist, and cultivate a state of serenity. In general, Thai massage sequences adhere to a predetermined structure, commencing with an opening and centering action, progressing to encompass a range of body parts, and culminating in a closing ritual.

Adaptations to Thai massage can be made to accommodate particular populations, including athletes and expectant women, while still ensuring the treatment remains effective and safe.

By incorporating additional therapeutic techniques, including deep tissue massage, Swedish massage, and yoga therapy, into Thai massage, a holistic and adaptable approach can be adopted to cater to the varied requirements of clients.

Thai massage, whether experienced as a practitioner or recipient, offers a distinctive and revitalizing encounter that transcends mere physical manipulation. It accomplishes this by integrating components of cultural tradition, energy equilibrium, mindfulness, and relaxation.

Prior to engaging in any type of bodywork or massage, it is advisable for individuals to engage in candid communication with their practitioners and carefully evaluate their personal health conditions.

THE END

www.ingramcontent.com/pod-product-compliance
Ingram Content Group UK Ltd.
Pitfield, Milton Keynes, MK11 3LW, UK
UKHW021408051025
8231UKWH00020B/207

9 798872 919292